Merry Fitness!! :)

JC

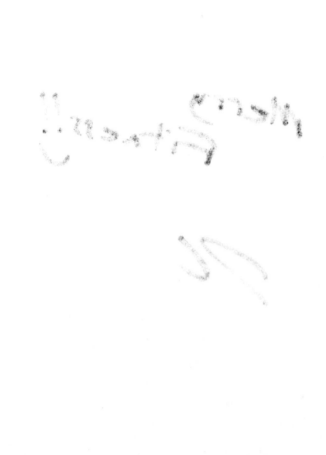

Kid Fitness
with Phillip and Natalie

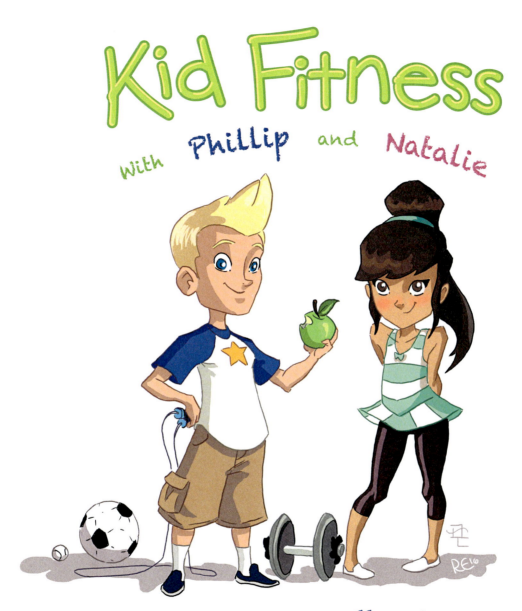

Created and Written by Jeff Caldwell Jr
Illustrated by Rachel Everett

Copyright © 2013 by Jeff Caldwell Jr.
www.kidfitnessbooks.com

This book is dedicated to all children and families around the world.

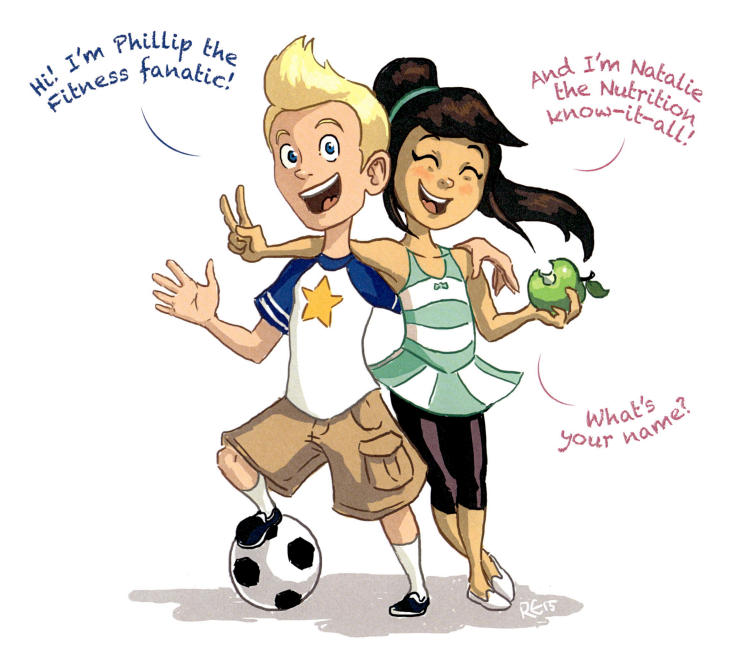

We love to keep our bodies and minds healthy and strong! To do this we do lots of super fun and important things!

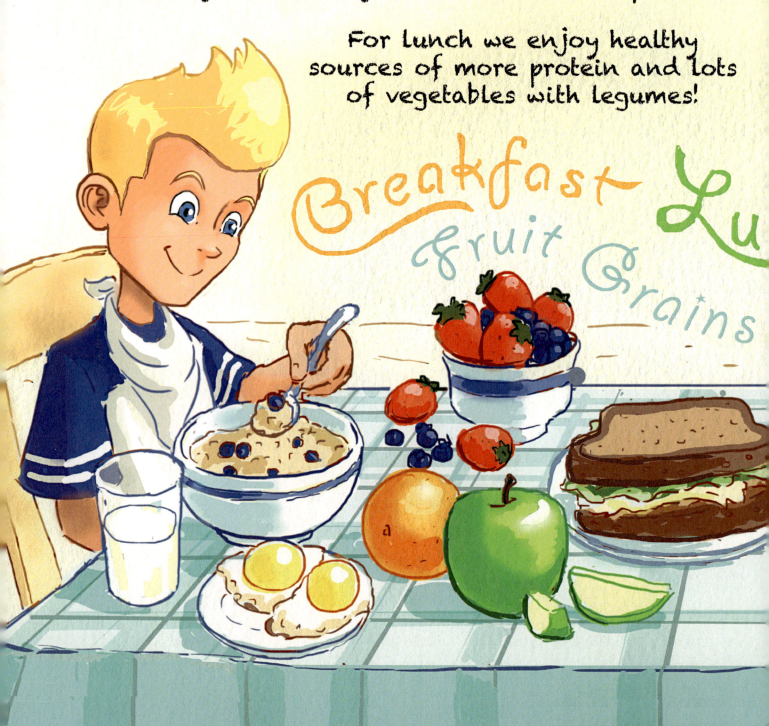

We start the day out right by eating foods with lots of natural energy like healthy grains, fruits, and proteins!

For lunch we enjoy healthy sources of more protein and lots of vegetables with legumes!

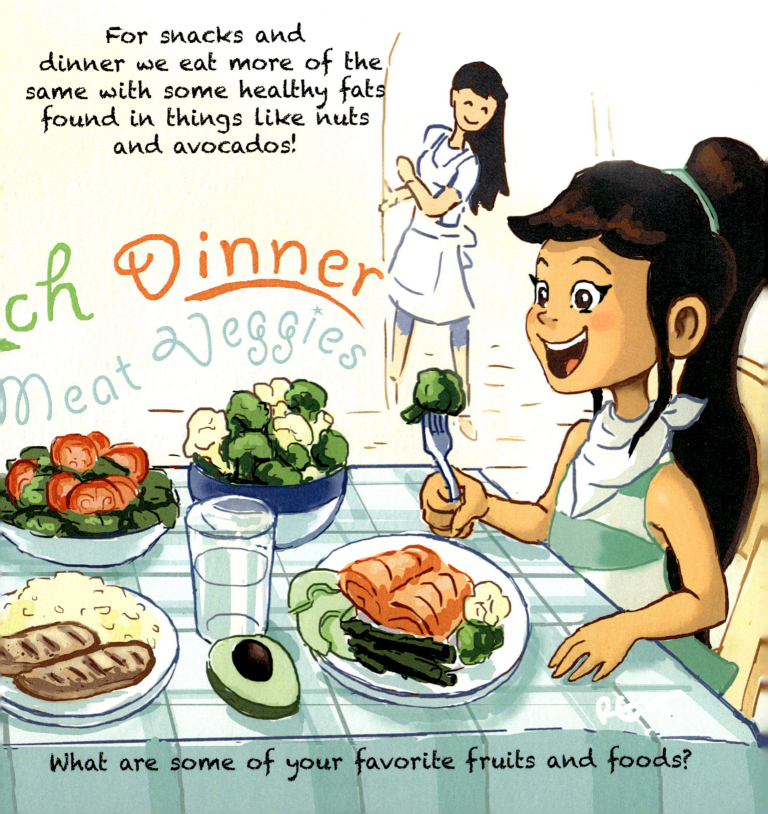

Eating foods with healthy vitamins and nutrients help us to grow strong all day and night long! When we become stronger, our energy lasts longer!

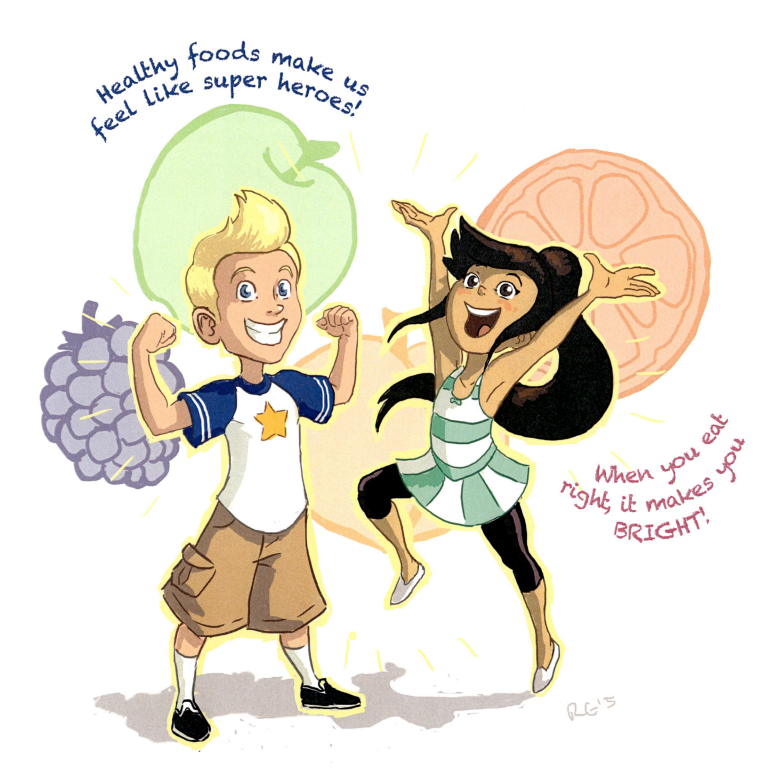

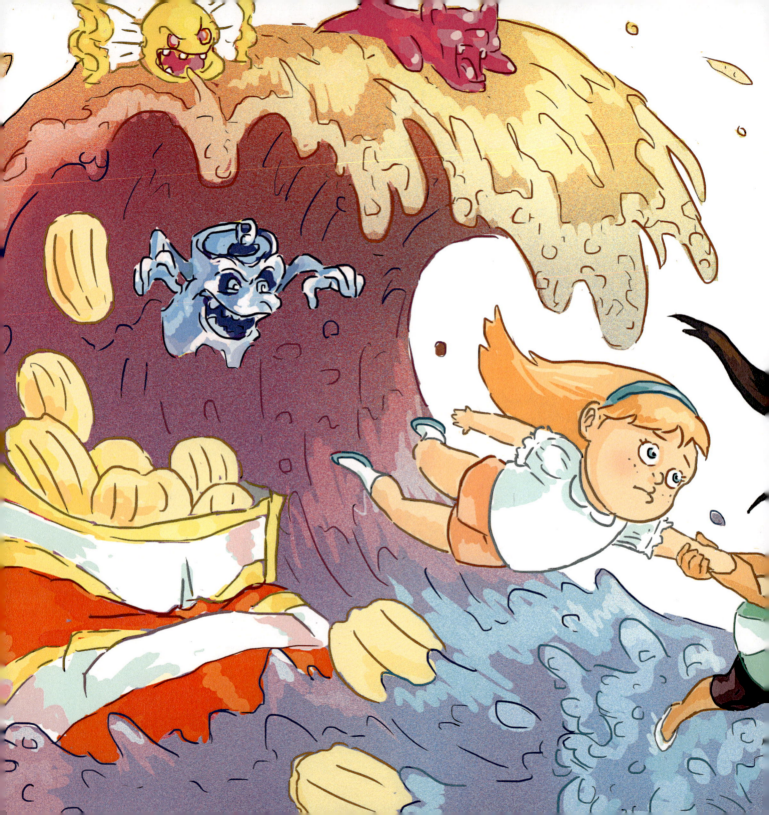

Bad sugars are what make us look and feel most unhealthy. Eating candy and junk foods and drinking soda cause us to feel slow, sleepy and sluggish. We often try our best to save our friends from the harmful effects of these poor choices.

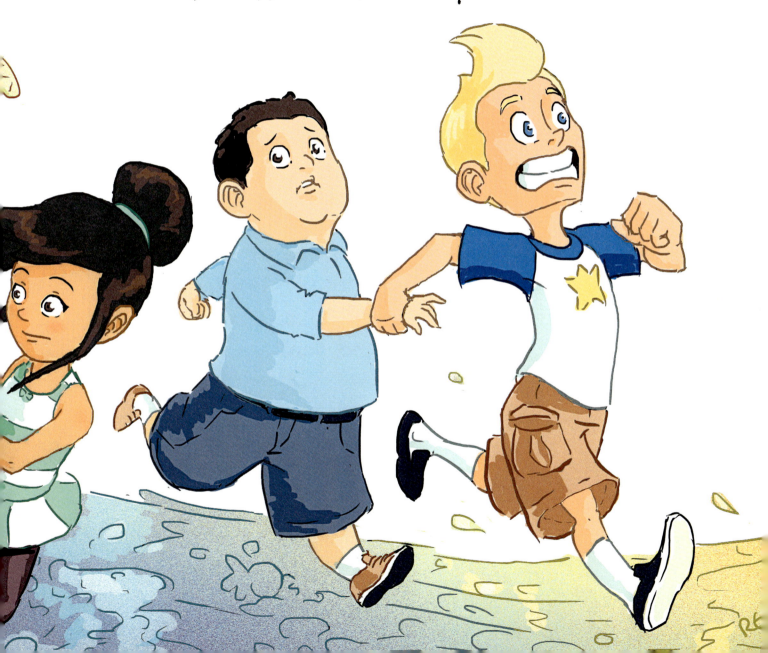

The next thing we do to be healthy and strong is to stay active every day! An active body helps our brains and feelings to stay positive and happy!

We like to participate in all kinds of activities like playing lots of different sports as well as exercise! They are so fun!!

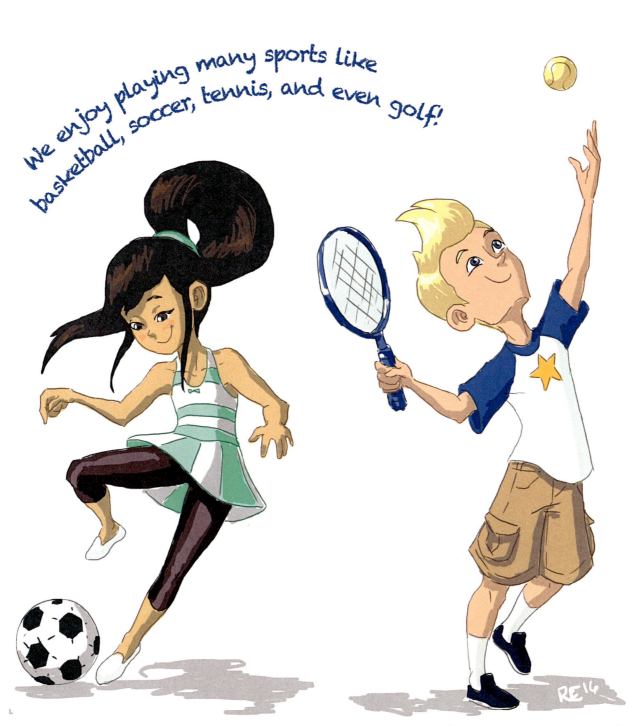

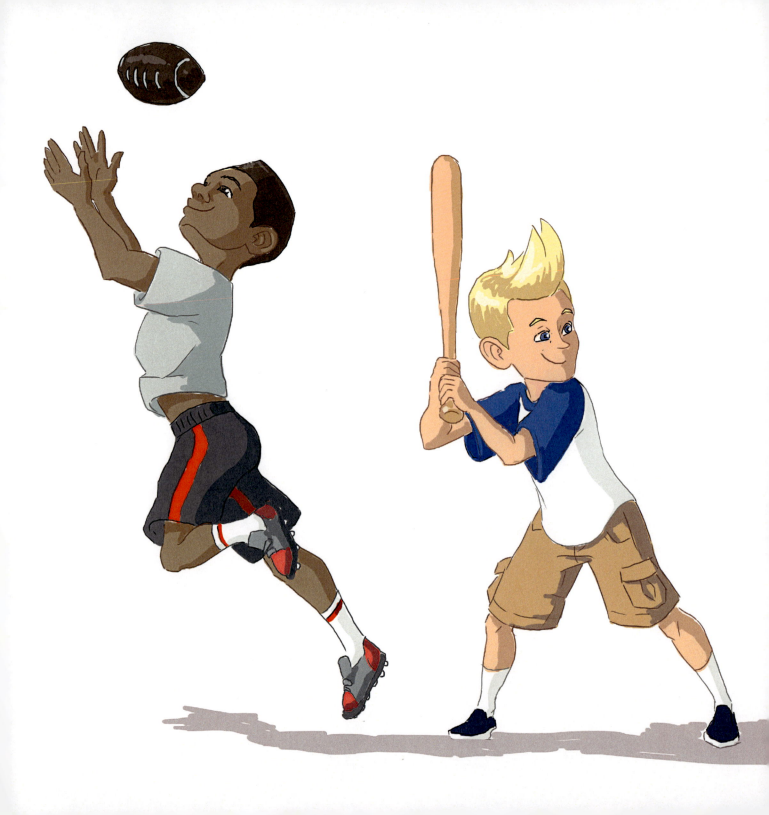

We also try playing other sports like baseball, bowling, football, and frisbee, plus more!

What is your favorite sport?!

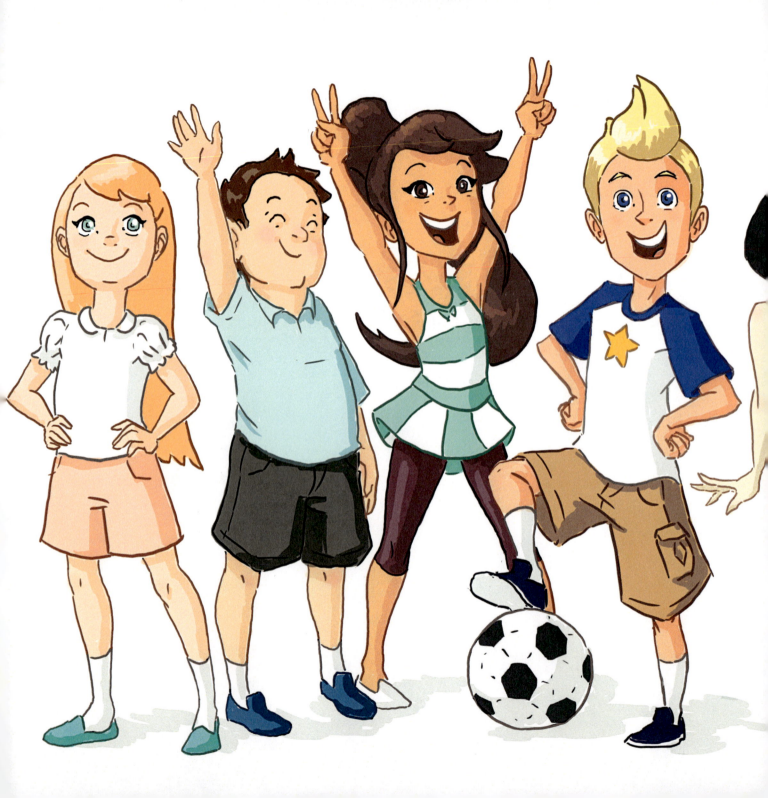

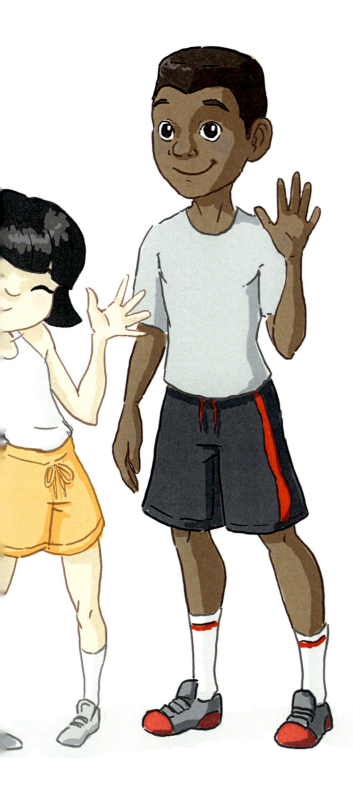

By playing sports, we learn to play as a team with our family and friends. We have the most fun when we get to play on the same teams!

We love our family and friends!

Do you ever get to play sports with your family?

For other exercise activities we like to jump rope, swim, jog, ride bikes, and even surf!

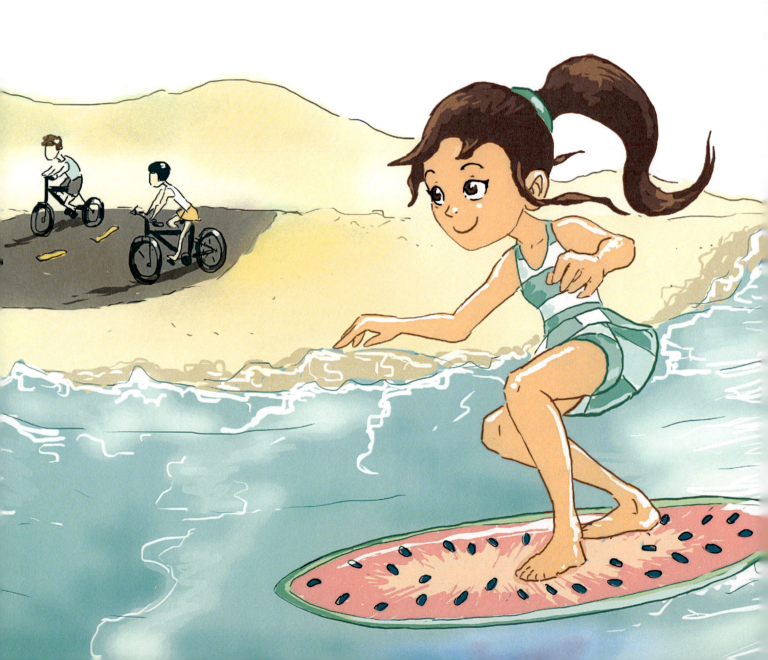

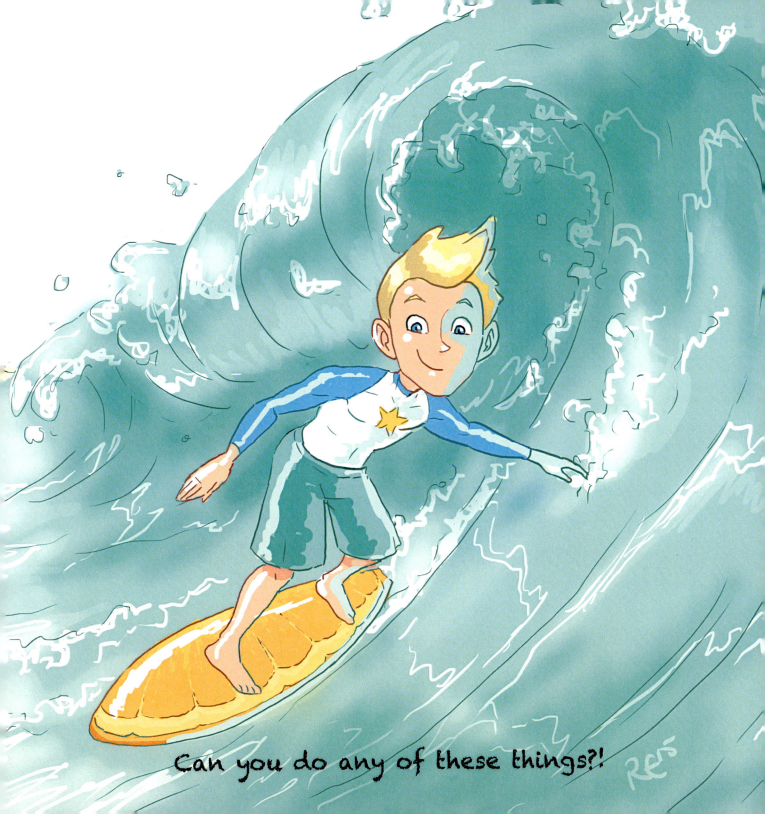

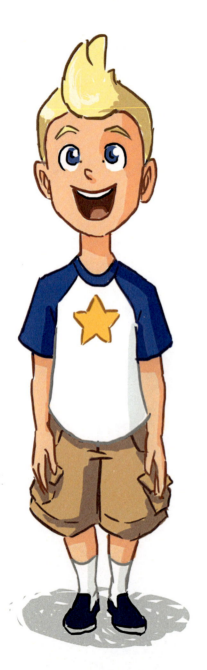
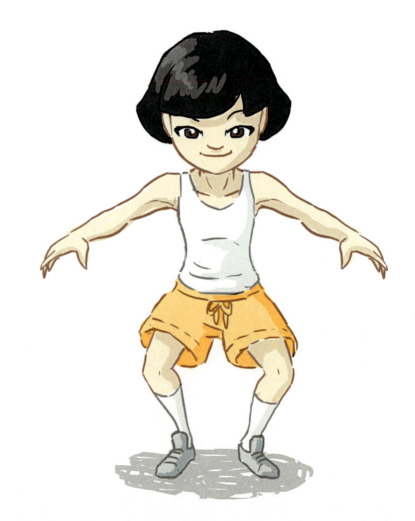

For more exercise we also do lots of jumping jacks!

Do you know how to do jumping jacks?

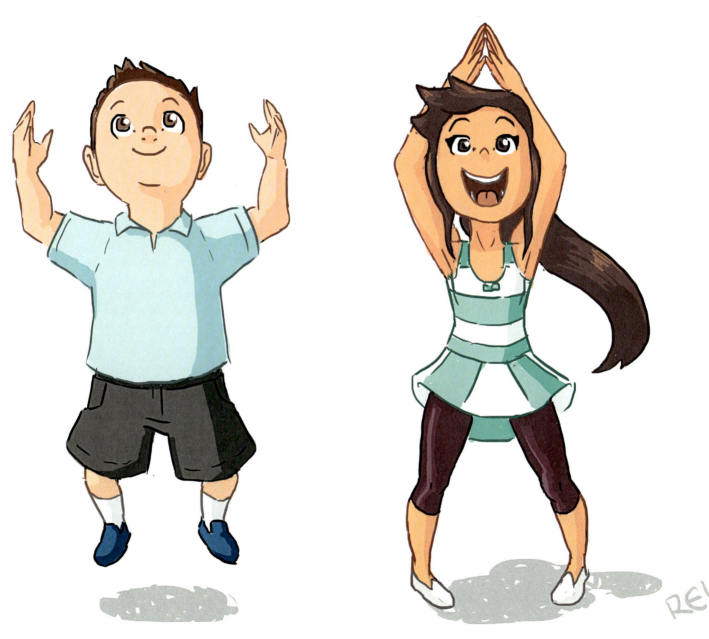

How many can you do in 1 minute?

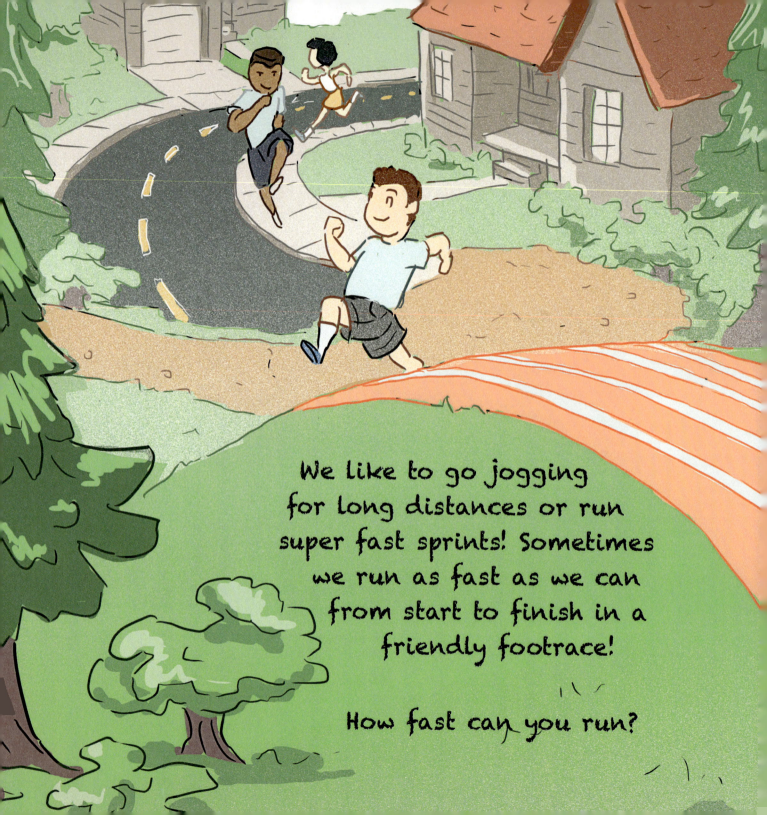

We like to go jogging for long distances or run super fast sprints! Sometimes we run as fast as we can from start to finish in a friendly footrace!

How fast can you run?

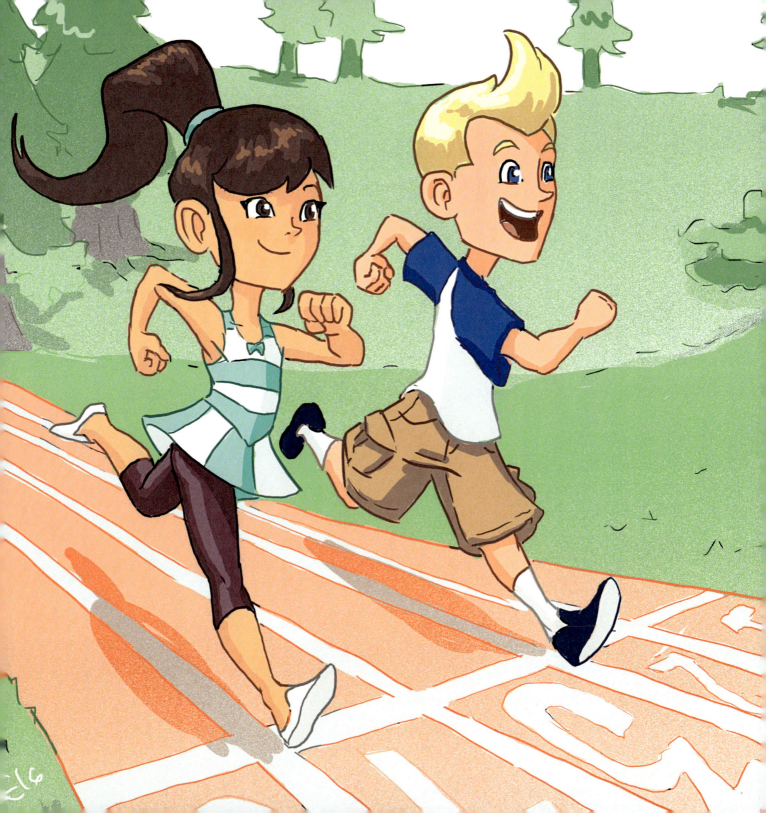

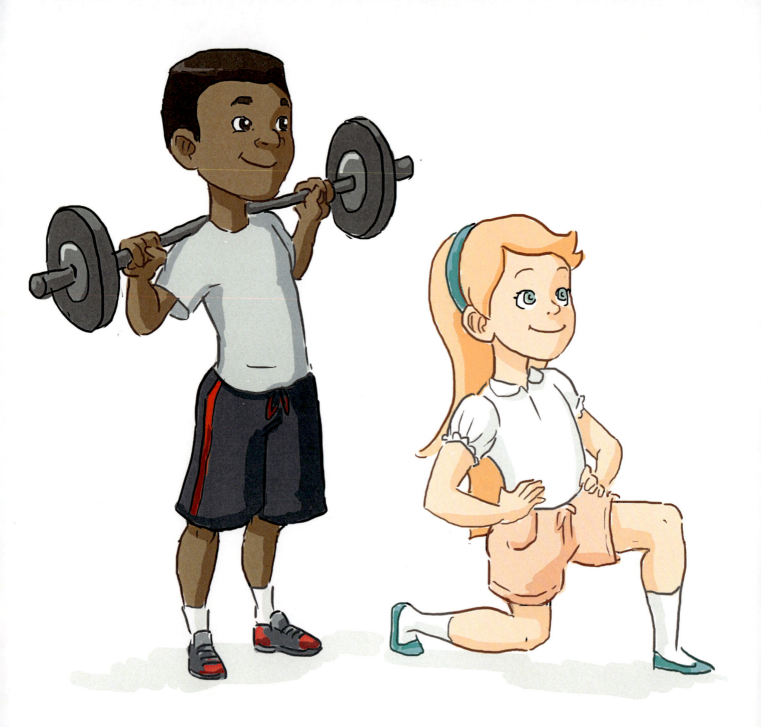

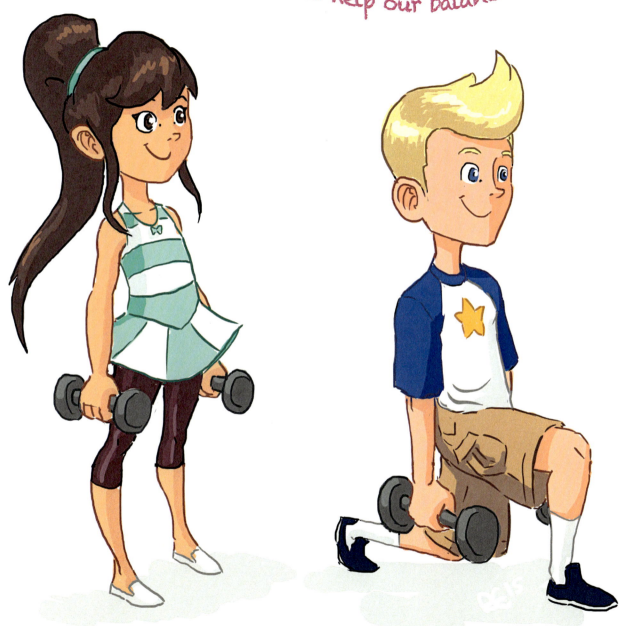

We do as many push-ups as we can! And sit-ups too! More than just a few!

How many can you do?

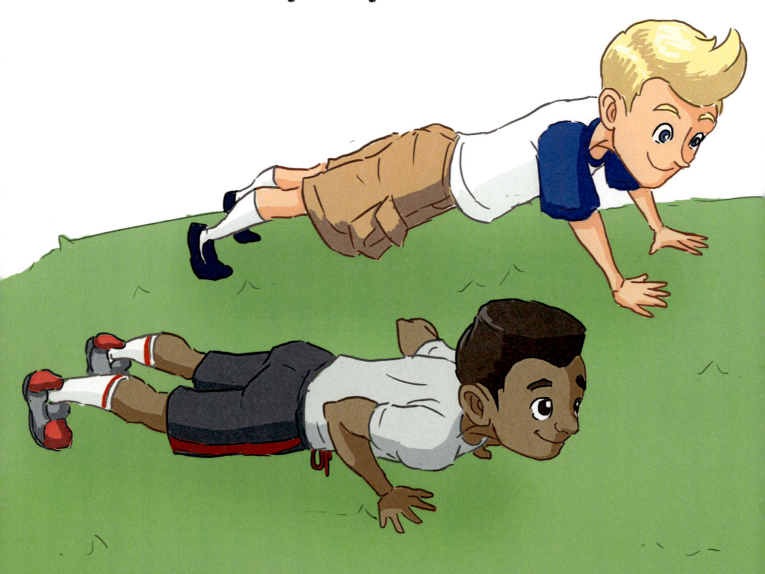

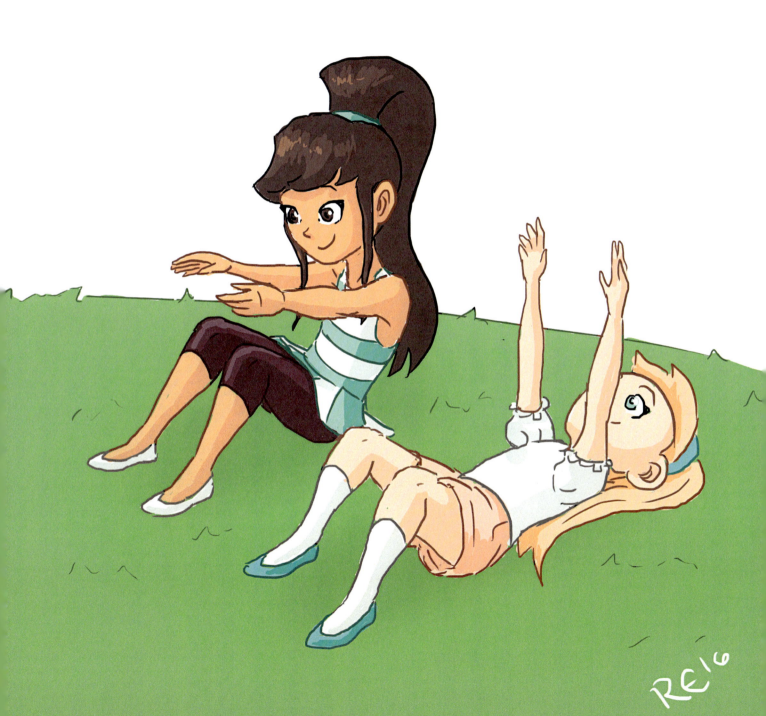

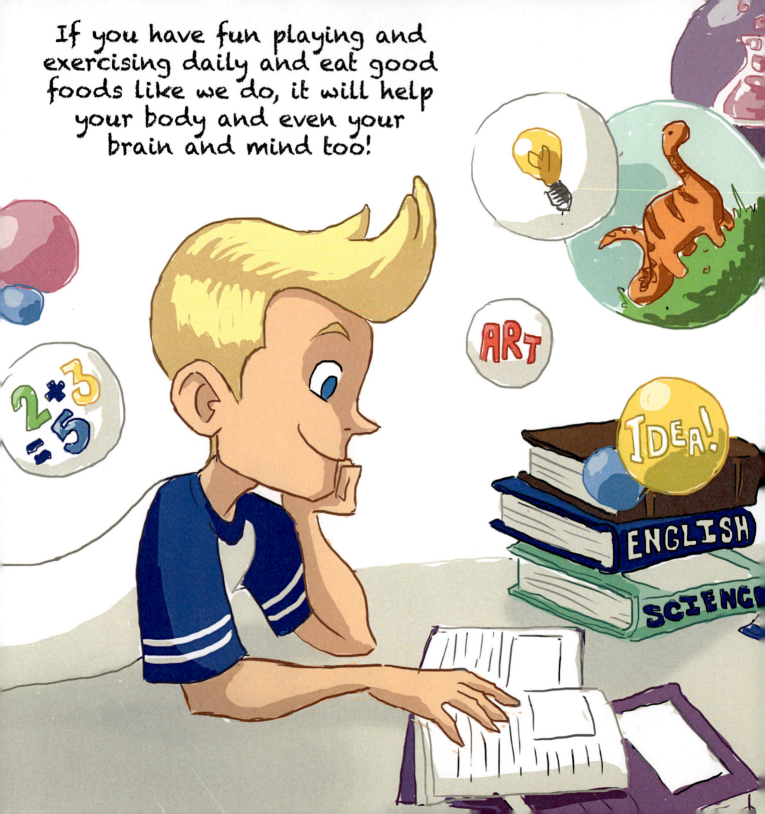

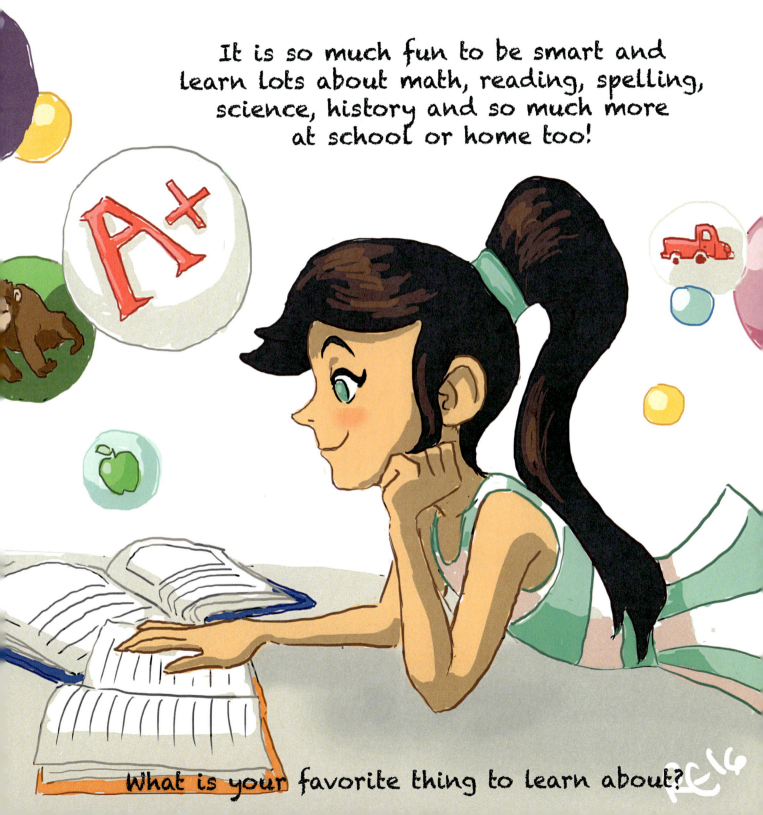

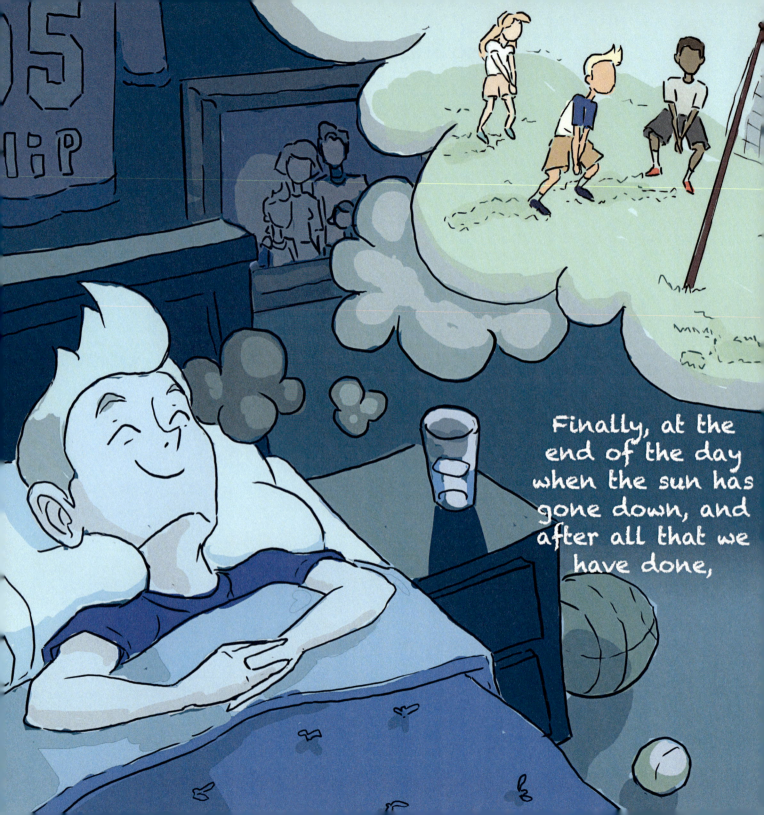

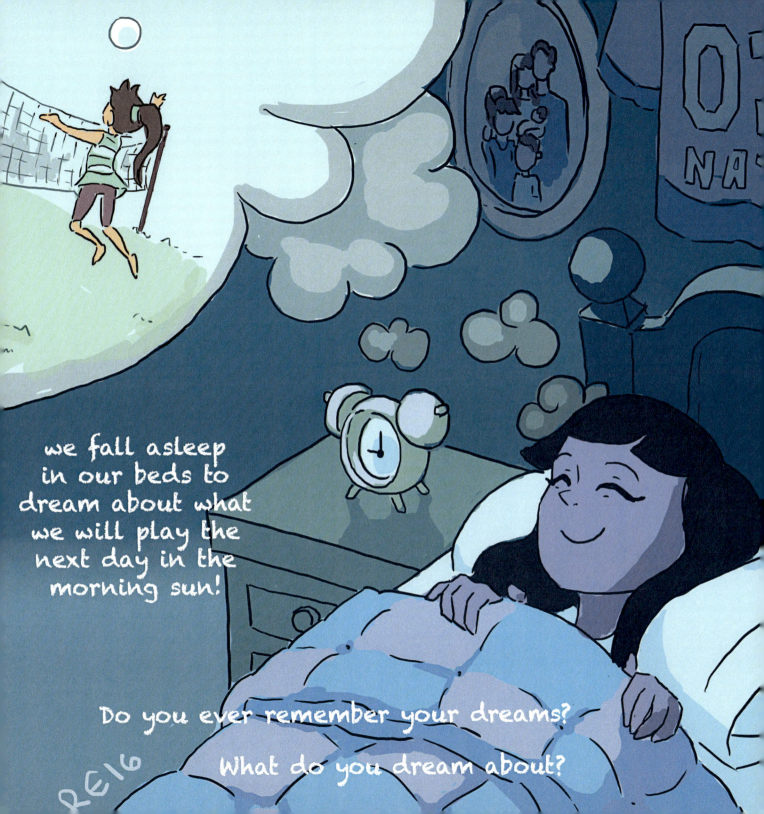

Getting lots of rest every night helps us reset and restore to full health and energy for the next day's activities. Sleeping for about 8-10 hours every night also helps us feel positive and happy about life!

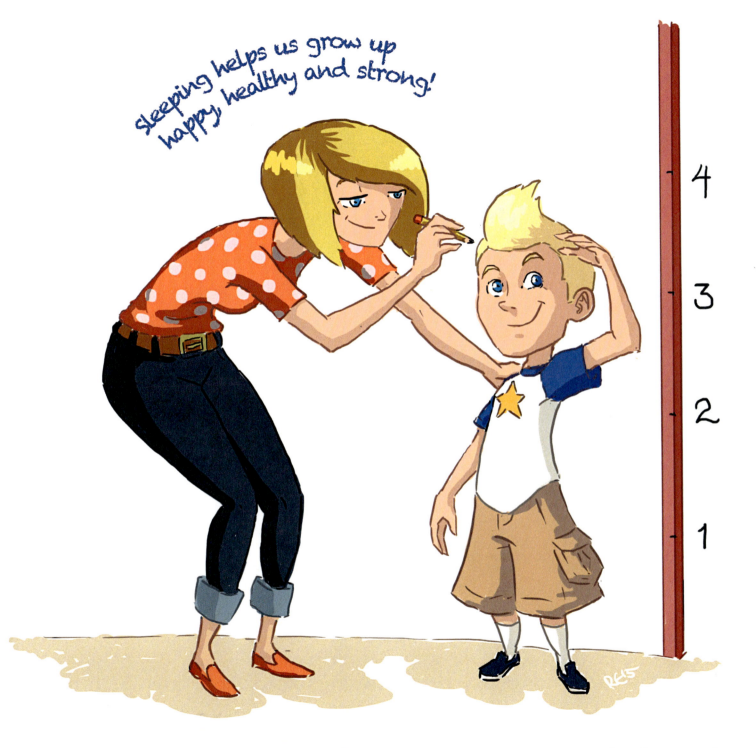

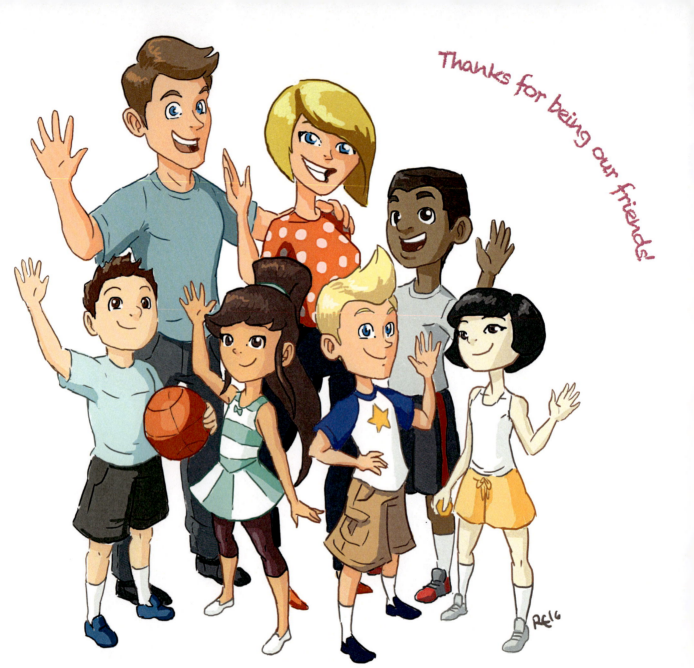

Thanks for being our friends!

Follow us and our healthy habits and you too will be happy, healthy, and strong, just like us! Join us again for some more Kid Fitness! You will have so much FUN!

Let's play again soon!

The End!

A special thanks to the following:

Jessika Lopez, for your stroke-of-genius encouragement to write this book.

Bryce Collins, for your original illustration work of Phillip and Natalie.

Lina and Siena Urquiza, for being my initial kid sounding boards.

Rachel Everett, for your incredible talent and professionalism in bringing the characters to life.

Cara Caldwell, for your undending support and love and for all your invaluable help to see this project come forth and for believing in me.

Tayler Christensen, for your website wizardry and ongoing consultations.

And you, the reader, for reading and buying my book!

I wish you all the very best health and happiness this life has to offer.

The People behind Kid Fitness

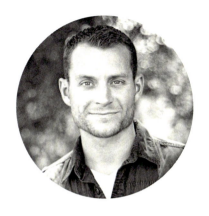

Jeff Caldwell Jr.
Creator/Author

Jeff Caldwell Jr is a College Certified Personal Trainer and has worked with a variety of clients from Hollywood to Utah since 2008. Growing up he was active and interested in many sports from baseball, basketball, soccer, wrestling, track & field, snow skiing and snowboarding to his young adult and adult ventures with tennis, golf, wake boarding, water skiing, surfing, mountain biking, cycling, softball, bowling, competitive running, and more.

He developed a love for staying active and fit from his father and step-father, who were athletic examples of regular exercise and weight training. As the oldest of 7 children, he has a natural passion for connecting with young children and teenagers. His all time favorite sport is baseball but loves any physical challenge or game. He regularly engages in exercise methods of circuit training, body-building, cross-fit, endurance training and most recently "Ninja Warrior" air sports.

Nutrition has always been an ongoing interest and passion for Jeff, as well as healthy cooking and eating. His life goal is to inspire and educate as many people as possible to live a happy and healthy lifestyle.

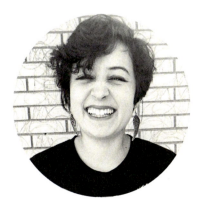

Rachel Everett
Illustrator

Rachel Everett has been drawing and telling stories since she was very little. She has always known she was going to be an artist when she grew up. She is the creator, writer, and illustrator of the independent comic book series 13 Light-Years Away, and has been doing freelance illustration since she was 15 years old.

Learn more at kidfitnessbooks.com

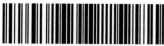

Made in the USA
San Bernardino, CA
27 August 2016